"THE HIDDEN TREASURE FOR PRACTITIONERS"

by

Reza Mostafavi

Table of Contents:

PREFACE

You might have experienced that you visit your first patient energetically and passionately in the morning but slowly the fatigue offsets your initial pep. Putting some conditions like anemia or hypothyroidism aside, this pattern is normal and can be magnified by the practitioner's physiological and psychological state. It's also largely dependent upon the type of clients you are dealing with every day. A cheerful patient with a sense of humor can make your day even as the last patient and a grumpy one can ruin your day just from the beginning.

But is there a solution to this problem? Is it possible to keep the pep until the last patient and reinforce the morning momentum?

When it comes to performance, most of the time, it's not a matter of time, it's a matter of pep.

There are endless amounts of books about time management but how many books talk about maintaining your physical and emotional energy during the day?

In this book, we address that question and offer the ultimate solution: self-hypnosis.

You will learn how to use the power of self-hypnosis or autosuggestion in your daily practice for yourself. You can also educate your patients.

One of the reasons I like Dave Elman, the great hypnotherapist is that he wanted the therapist himself to take advantage of hypnotherapy first. This "Pay yourself first attitude" about hypnotherapy attracted me a while ago. If hypnotherapy is an effective tool, why not to use it for yourself as a therapist first?

This book is about practical and pragmatic solutions. I explain the theoretical aspect of hypnosis briefly in this manuscript. If this is your first encounter with hypnosis, suggestions, and metaphors, my aim is to speak to both beginners and seasoned hypnotherapists by asking myself:

"Will this material teach me how to sustain the peppiness all day long?".

After reading this book, and applying it in your daily routine, not only will you have more energy during the day, you will also have more time as a result of this increased energy. The added benefit of this manuscript will provide you with a shield to protect yourself against the unwanted negativity you absorb from your patients. This phenomenon is called compassion fatigue.

Devote this time to learn about hypnosis for you and help your patients and clients enjoy the benefits of hypnosis as you do!

My mission is to introduce the evidence-based hypnotherapy as a great therapeutic modality. My job is to clear the wrong perceptions about hypnosis and introduce that as a strong clinically proved approach rather than a mystical or supernatural entity.

Please send me your feedback and help me to optimize this book in future revisions.

You can find more information on my website:

www.treata.ca

Chapter One: An introduction to Suggestions and Metaphors

We have all experienced spontaneous trance throughout our lives. Some of us are more talented when it comes to those experiences - in other words more innate - and some of us experience that dissociation state less often. So, we all have experienced spontaneous self-hypnosis to some degree. The general objective of hypnotherapy is:

1-to make these trance experiences intentional.

and

2-Use them for a specific purpose through an agenda.

There are other platforms like yoga, meditation and mindfulness to experience trance. However, the issue with other platforms in a clinical setting is the lack of agenda. In a therapeutic setting, the whole point of entering a trance state is to take advantage of a hyper-suggestibility state which is observed during the trance. The content – called suggestions – are designed specifically and carefully and are the backbone of the whole process and ultimate agenda. There is neither nothing wrong with having a session without an agenda nor using meditation or yoga as a therapy but I'm not a fan of that. Because I believe when you get into trance, you need to utilize it into the fullest through "suggestions".

Before we start to apply self-hypnosis to keep our pep and momentum during the day, we need to know a little bit about hypnosis.

One way (which is not necessarily the best way) to start discovering about an entity is to define it. The problem is that there is no consensus about the definition of hypnosis! Different definitions of hypnosis have caused the emerging of different schools of thought in hypnotherapy. To prevent from being stuck at the beginning, we will stick to the definition of American Society of Clinical Hypnosis in this manuscript:

Clinical hypnosis is an altered state of awareness, perception or consciousness that is used, by licensed and trained doctors or masters prepared individuals, for treating a psychological or physical problem. It is a highly relaxed state.

(https://www.asch.net/Public/GeneralInfoonHypnosis/FAQsAboutHypnosis.aspx)

Under hypnosis, the subjects are more receptive to suggestions and this fact makes hypnosis a great platform for making some psychological or physiological changes. There are different phases in hypnosis including induction, deepening, suggestions, and termination. The desired change is suggested in "suggestion phase".

There are a lot of questions about the mechanism of hypnosis and we don't know how it exactly works and why suggestions can make even some physiological changes.

Having said that, there is a lot of evidence in clinical studies (many are randomized double-blind clinical trials with the highest levels of evidence) showing that hypnosis leads to sustainable results. New advances in brain imaging like f MRI (Functional Magnetic Resonance Imaging) and

PET Scan (Positive Emission Tomography) has provided us with a great understanding of the neuroscientific basis of hypnosis during the recent years.

In terms of the mechanism of hypnosis, the model I resonated with is the "metacognition game model".

Metacognition is a cognition about another cognition. In other words, an insight about the cognition. For example, you may have back pain. Simultaneously, you understand and acknowledge that you have that pain (you have an insight – which is a more complex cognition – about that pain). The latter is a metacognition which is much more sophisticated comparing to the primary cognition and is associated with a lot of memories and past experiences. We may categorize a lot of affective components of pain as metacognition.

A lot of varieties you see among people in terms of pain threshold are related to different metacognitions created over a similar cognition rather than personal anatomical or physiological variations.

There is no clear cut-off point between cognition and metacognition and it makes a safe sense to say they are 2 extremes of a spectrum in practice.

Another example of metacognition is when you don't remember the name of a famous actor or actress and after a while, of struggling, (specially for those who suffer from OCD, that can be torture!) you remember it. The name of the actor or actress is a cognition and the fact that you know the name (but for some reason you don't remember it) is a metacognition.

In this model, hypnosis is a metacognition game. Hypnosis manipulates the meta-cognition, so the cognitions are felt in a modified, attenuated, accentuated or even reversed (opposite) way. Bypassing the critical factor is the first step in this process and that happens when the subject trusts the therapist in terms of both integrity and competence. The subject voluntarily suspends the critical judgment – up to a certain level – to take advantage of hypnosis.

I've found the metacognition game the best convincing model for myself, as a result, I'm a little bit hesitant to use hypnosis as sole anesthesia particularly with acute pain. The reason for this is when I use hypnosis as the sole anesthesia, I feel the patient is experiencing the pain in another level while the patient is completely relaxed and calm. In other words, I suspect that despite the fact the metacognition shows no sign of suffering, at the cognition level – which is masked under the power of metacognition – the pain is felt unconsciously. That's why I think hypnosis should be used in conjunction with other modalities when it comes to pain management. It's similar to an anesthesiologist who still needs to use opioids as the painkiller even though the patient is under general anesthesia. Otherwise, tachycardia or high blood pressure will interfere with the normal course of operation.

Every Hypnosis is Self-Hypnosis

This is crucial to understand that every hypnosis is self-hypnosis and as a result, the role of the hypnotherapist is as facilitator or as Dave Elman says: operator. Stage hypnotists and movies have a tendency to illustrate the exact opposite image for commercial purposes. A beginner hypnotherapist may get into this delusional trap after seeing the power of hypnotherapy at the beginning.

Every hypnotherapy plan has a transition phase or weaning phase to remove the hypnotherapist from the equilibrium and keep the patient or subject independent. This transition phase is different in different people and different situations. As a rule of thumb, the 6th session is a good time to start educating the patient about self-hypnosis. Having said that, some patients are ready for self-hypnosis in the first session and some are not open to it even after 20 sessions.

There are 2 main methods to conduct the self-hypnosis: Anchoring & Regular hypnotic induction.

In anchoring, a hypnotherapist hypnotizes you and when you are in a deep trance, you will be conditioned to a "cue". For example, in a deep trance, the hypnotist will tell you: "Whenever you sit on this comfortable chair and take 3 deep breaths, you get back to this depth of trance". This Cue should be unique and specific enough.

The other method is making suggestions to yourself just as you would for your subject for hypnosis induction.

In this book, we are focusing on the 2nd method. However, you may ask your colleague or hypnotherapist to use the anchoring method for you and then apply the suggestions we will discuss later, in this book.

(If you are a psychologist using psychoanalysis and psychodynamic, transference is another factor dictating the number of sessions needed. However, I haven't seen any value in any form of transference despite the emphasis of Sigmund Freud and Carl Jung on that but it's up to you to decide)

Chapter Two: Induction & Deepening

The rate-limiting step in hypnosis induction is bypassing the critical judgment.

One of the best techniques to induce hypnosis for yourself is "pretending". This technique is primarily used by Dave Elman. We have modified the technique a little bit and you can alter it yourself as well based on your creativity once you understand the concept and its principles.

I usually use the pretending technique for patients who resist hypnosis. This resistance is unconscious and unintentional most of the times. It also may work if the subject is resisting intentionally. But the easier way for conscious resistant is to clarify that hypnosis is not a good option for the subject.

I start the process by asking them to watch a video of a person who is under hypnosis (I send the video to them in advance). Then I ask them to pretend they are hypnotized by mimicking the subject's facial expressions and gestures. Catalepsy (Muscular rigidity) is a part of the video. It's like role-playing (This approach is sometimes like psychodrama or dramatherapy while the subject is involved in theatre or ritual). I ask the subject to conduct the role-playing "as real" as I can't differentiate between him/her pretending and the actual hypnotized subject.

It may seem that this technique is more suitable for people who are extroverts. Paradoxically, based on my experience, the subjects who are more introverted are as engaged as the extroverts in the game. Maybe the reason is they find a secure non-verbal platform to communicate.

In the last phase, I want them to open their eyes and relax. I apply fractionation in this phase. We will discuss fractionation later on. Then I ask them to pretend again so well that this time even him/herself can't differentiate! Even if they could watch themselves objectively as an external observer, they could not see they are pretending. This helps a lot of people – even those who are resisting – to get into trance smoothly.

After the trance is induced, the next step is to deepen the trance. The simplest way to do that is using the fractionation technique.

Hypnotists – during the early years of using hypnosis - realized that the first session is usually the lightest trance in an individual and gradually the trance would get deeper in the following sessions. So, they minimized the intervals between the sessions and observed the deepening trend still exists. They also realized that they can decrease the intervals into seconds and the trend still exists. So, when the trance is induced, if you ask the subject to open their eyes for a few seconds and then close them, it deepens the trance significantly. Hypnotherapists use this technique a lot and you can also do so.

Some subjects who are more hypnotizable may be unable to open their eyes and you may just see slight eye flutters or even nothing. It can still be effective in deepening the trance, even though the subject is unable to open the eyes.

The fractionation technique is also a great opportunity to estimate how deep the trance already is. When the subject opens the eyes, you can watch how congested the sclera is and how much the lacrimal glands are secreting. Soon, we will discuss the 5 signs of hypnosis.

Most induction techniques are deepening techniques as well and vise versa. You can even start the induction by fractionation. For example, you may say:

"I will start counting from 1 to 20 and you will open your eyes with odd numbers and close your eyes with even numbers…"

To make it more effective you can pause on even numbers a little bit longer.

When hypnosis is deep enough, you might start the suggestions. We will discuss the suggestions in the next chapter. Now, we will discuss 5 signs of hypnotic state mentioned by Dave Elman. You can use the following signs to watch if hypnosis is induced and if it is deep enough to go to the next step which might be suggestions.

ELMAN 5 SIGNS OF HYPNOSIS

Dave Elman mentions 5 signs to check if the patient is hypnotized or not. While they are not set in stone these signs are great guidelines to watch for during the induction and deepening of trance.

The first one is body warmth. You can easily shake hand with your clients, so you will get a sense of his or her body temperature.

The second one is eyelid fluttering while the subject is closing the eyes.

The third is the lacrimation increases.

The forth is the sclera gets congested and pinkish.

And fifth, the eyeballs go up.

Anchoring:

Anchoring is like conditioning. The subject gets conditioned to a "cue" or an "anchor" to reach a deeper level of hypnosis .

Previously, we mentioned you may use anchoring if you are hypnotized by another person. It does not mean you can't use it if you start self-hypnosis from scratch. You can save time for subsequent sessions if you condition yourself with an "anchor" whenever you feel you are deep enough in trance. You might suggest to yourself:

"Now, Next time when You I'm sitting in this comfortable chair and I take 3 deep breaths, I will get to this depth of trance I am experiencing now. I take my time and enjoy my deep trance."

You can even practice the "cue":

"You can imagine -everybody can imagine – you are awake, and you are practicing self-hypnosis…"

It's like a hypnosis over hypnosis. Dave Elman calls this "compounding of suggestions".

"Imagery techniques" and "sensory awareness" are not only induction techniques but also great deepening techniques. The Elevator metaphor is a great method to deepen the trance. You may say to your subject or yourself:

"Now imagine you are in an elevator and the elevator is going down. There are 10 levels. In each level, you take a deep breath and you become deeper and deeper. I don't know how fast the elevator is going down and to be honest, you don't know as well; but your unconscious mind knows exactly how fast the elevator is going down. Don't be in a rush. Take your time. Watch the elevator going down and you become deeper and deeper. Breathe in each level and enjoy your trance…"

You may use the staircase metaphor as an alternative to the elevator. If the patient has difficulty with movement – for example due to knee arthrosis – don't use this metaphor because it may interfere with the imagination and the patient may feel knee pain!

Imagination is not only an induction but also a deepening technique. One of the common scenarios is the image of a beautiful beach on a sunny day. The more of our 5 senses that are involved in the imagination, the more effective the deepening technique will be.

One of the other effective imagery techniques to deepen

trance is to imagine a wheel on the horizon with small round lights in the middle of the spokes.

"The wheel starts spinning firstly slowly and then faster and the lights create a light circle in the air…"

Chapter Three: Suggestions

Suggestions and metaphors are the core of hypnotherapy. The content of this phase which should be selected carefully is what makes you feel as peppy as when you started the day.

This is the phase, where the critical judgment (factor) is relaxed and you are open and receptive to suggestions. Sometimes the metaphors are stronger rather than direct suggestions. For example, when you get to the appropriate level of trance, you may simply suggest to yourself that you are as peppy as when visiting the first patients. You may close your eyes for a few seconds and remember the first few patients during the day.

The alternative to direct suggestion is a metaphor. For example, you may imagine you are taking a shower and washing out all the tiredness and stress.

You may also feel a headache during the day. You can simply use an autosuggestion and imagine your right hand is getting numb. Then you may suggest to yourself that – not now – but whenever your right-hand touches your head (or any other part of your body), the feeling you have goes away. Preferably avoid using the word "pain".

Based on your medical knowledge, this may seem ridiculous outside the trance. In trance, even in a light one, you are much more receptive to autosuggestions. The critical faculty may be suspended partially, and you may still see a kind of rediculessness in the game, but it does not mean you stop responding to the suggestions and that's why you are surprised. It's a good idea to use these moments of surprise as a "convincer" to paralyze the critical faculty more and make the trance deeper. These convincers are used quite often in hypnotherapy to leverage the momentum of deepening of the hypnosis.

As mentioned, sometimes, the use of metaphors is stronger than direct suggestions. Another example of that – as an alternative to direct suggestion - is to imagine it's in the morning and you are taking the shower and washing out all the tiredness down into the drain.

We will get back to this metaphor again when discussing compassion fatigue and ways to overcome that.

One of the other ways to use autosuggestions in your daily practice is to increase focus and concentration particularly at the end of the day. A few sentences about concentration can make a huge difference. An equivalent metaphor – like the imagination of a pinpoint focus on sunlight through a magnifier – can have the same strength.

Chapter Four: Termination

In a therapeutic approach, the termination is very important. Physiologically, you should return the subject into pre-hypnosis state before the sessions end. It's not wise to leave the patient under generalized muscle relaxation and simply ask to open the eyes.

Having said that, when you use hypnosis for yourself in a clinical setting, you may decide not to terminate that completely. That will be more applicable if you use hypnosis mainly for concentration on your job. The truth is, if you love your job, you get into a trance state whenever you concentrate on it. Hypnosis is a triad of concentration, suggestibility, and dissociation in varying degrees.

To have an idea about "waking hypnosis", I give you an example. You may have experienced watching your favorite movie or TV series and becoming unable to hear the sounds around you. Your attention is focusing on some selected auditory inputs and filters out all other sounds and assumes them as noises. While you are starring at the screen, you may not hear an offer for a tea or coffee. In these circumstances, the spontaneous hypnosis starts with an attentive concentration and that leads to a dissociation from the environment. If you are experiencing it a lot, it is a sign of high hypnotizablity. If this is the case, you should be very mindful about your self-talks because you are very receptive to them particularly when experiencing some episodes of spontaneous trance.

However, even if you love your job, sometimes your workload can become too much and that's when hypnosis and autosuggestion is a perfect fit to get the momentum back.

It's essentially important not to rush to driving right after experiencing a deep trance. It is also common sense as you never jump behind the wheel after waking up early in the morning! It's pretty much the same.

Reverse suggestions to return the physiology into the pre-suggestion state is important in hypnodontics (hypnosis in dentistry). We should never leave a patient numb after applying anesthesia with hypnosis. Bleeding control is also common in hypnodontics. We should not forget to make some suggestions to return the bleeding tendency as it was before terminating the trance.

In a clinical setting, it's important to provide at least 10 minutes for the patient to share their hypnosis experience. That's a valuable opportunity for the clinician to discover great clues about the patient and modify the approach accordingly. My humble advice is Never lose that brilliant opportunity after hypnosis termination.

The role of "Post-termination" discussion is more valuable in some highly hypnotizable subjects. Generally, we can categorize highly hypnotizable subjects in 2 large categories:

1-Imaginative

2-Dissociative

The former's experience is full of vivid imagination and creativity while the later's trance is more about detachment from the environment. In the dissociative type of the highly hypnotizable patient, they don't remember the conversation with the therapist and the communication channel between the two is minimal. The only time to communicate the suggestions in these subjects is right before or very shortly after the trance.

If you do have time, you may decide to hypnotize the subject again right after the conversation to achieve your therapeutic goals.

Chapter Five: Make the pep contagious: "Pacing & Leading"

We sometimes forget how strong our words are, how deep we interact with deep language structures and how easy a body gesture or facial expression can make all the difference. I remember participating in a panel discussion of people using a substance and one of them said: "Sometimes it takes a smile to save a life". I will also add: "Sometimes it's simply saying: "I care about you" to save a life.

Not only can you use autosuggestion to stay peppy all day long, but you may also transfer that to your clients as a gift. You can also share this gift with your colleagues and enjoy the synergistic vibe in the team.

The technique we discuss here is truism & "pacing and leading" which are practical conversational (or covert) techniques. Whenever I use the term covert hypnosis, some of my colleagues roll their eyes and look at me skeptically. I believe that there is a place for using covert hypnosis as long as you use it as an honest persuasive technique and not as a deceptive trick.

The truism is starting the conversation by emphasizing on obvious facts (like describing the weather) and bypassing the critical judgment by normal fatigue. When the critical faculty receives obvious facts, it gets numb and then you can make your suggestions verbally or through your body language to induce relaxation and stillness into your client.

Although this process is continuous and there is no separation, for the sake of simplicity we categorize it as pacing, synchronization and leading. To monitor when is the best time to start suggestions (in another word detecting the signs of synchronization) you may monitor your client for example by checking his or her pulse rate and simultaneously and watch for any possible catalepsy.

Catalepsy is a neurological condition known as muscular rigidity. It's a sign of hypnotizablity and readiness to enter into a suggestible state. If you remember the signs of trance from chapter 2, body warmth, eye fluttering, excessive lacrimation, congested sclera and eye roll, these are great indicators of trance even in a conversational context. When you see your patient is showing signs of hypnosis, you may start smiling and suggest a few positive sentences about energy and happiness or whatever suggestion the subject needs.

"Pacing and leading" is pretty much like the truism. The only difference is instead of focusing on obvious facts at the beginning, you try to mimic the subjects body language and facial expression. This should be gradual, subtle and artistic rather than an artificial bold reflex. Imagine your last client steps into your office grumpy and tired. Your facial expression does not show you are also grumpy because that's against your larger goal! The better alternative is to try to mimic the client's pattern of respiration. That's a very strong way for the pacing phase.

You may find it hard at the beginning but after a while, you will become unconsciously competent in it and it becomes a part of you. I have also tried to be grumpy (as the pacing phase) with a grumpy client and most of the time it works. You have to be careful though because sometimes it affects your rapport with the patient right at the beginning. If you want to try that (starting grumpy with a grumpy client!), my advice is to be sure in advance that your client is suggestible enough. Never try this for a new patient.

The leading phase can be merged with your therapy itself particularly if the chief complaint has a portion of the psychosomatic element which is the case much of the time. Sometimes this simple maneuver ("pacing and leading") helps you get rid of a lot of investigation to rule out the medical differential diagnoses of a psychosomatic complaint.

Chapter Six: Wash out the negativities absorbed from your clients (Compassion Fatigue)

Compassion Fatigue or Secondary Traumatic Stress (STS) is common amongst healthcare professionals and even lawyers. These professionals are exposed to a lot of negativity all day long and if they don't have a plan to protect themselves, they will experience anxiety, depression and compassion fatigue down the road. The professional may also become desensitized and loses the ability to connect to his/her clients and it affects the rapport with the clients.

Hypnosis is not only a great way to keep the pep during the day, but it is also like a bulletproof jacket against negativities around the professional. The metaphor I like the most, in this case, is the imagination of taking a shower:

The professional – during the break or at the end of the day – induces a quick and light self-hypnosis and imagines taking a shower and washing out all the negative feelings absorbed during the day down to the drain. If the subject is able to imagine but there is a resistance to washing out the negativities, changing the picture in mind can help a lot.

The subject may imagine zooming in or out of the image, changing the color and making it black and white and watch how it affects the feeling. It's an example of one of the applications of N.L.P (Neuro Linguistic Programming) in hypnosis. I had a client who was able to imagine washing all the negativities down to the drain.

However, she reported seeing a kind of "mold" on her face preventing her from cleaning it. She started applying N.L.P to the picture and was able to get rid of that difficulty.

(The strange thing was the patient reported an episode of skin hypersensitivity in that facial area 2 days later which was self-limiting).

Sometimes you have the luxury of taking a shower during your workday. If so, a combination of this metaphor with a real shower is so synergistic. Showers are the only places in our lives which are not occupied by technology (Yet!) because our cell phones are not still waterproof enough. So, that haven is a great place to use autosuggestions without any distraction.

If you get into the habit of using shower time for autosuggestion, you will gift yourself a couple of productive hours during the day.

Try to use that opportunity because it won't last long and Google, Apple and Samsung will ruin that safe place very soon.

Chapter Seven: Expand the applications

Well, if hypnosis is efficient for yourself, why not to use it for your clients?

No matter what kind of health care professional you are, you can always use hypnotherapy in your practice. Hypnosis is a strong therapeutic modality when it comes to medical conditions, cancer, low self-esteem, acute and chronic pains, anxiety and psychological problems, sleep disorders, obesity and eating disorders, habit disorders, sexual dysfunction and countless other indications.

I think by now you have a great overall understanding of hypnotherapy.

Maybe the best resource to learn more about hypnotherapy is American Society of Clinical Hypnosis:

www.asch.com

I have created a FREE online course called "Hypnosis First Look":

http://hfl.treata.ca

For over 10 years, I have read different schools of thoughts in hypnosis, applied them in my practice, optimized the process and summarized it for you in this course.